Delectable

Lectin-Free Recipes

Breakfast, Lunch, Dinner and Dessert
Meals for Gut Health, Weight Loss, and that
Peak Body you Desire

Ainsley Neal

-Table of Content-

–Tofu and Vegetable Stir-Fry–

✓ Dinner!

–Lemon-Baked Chicken Thighs–
–Spaghetti Squash Bolognese–
–Grilled salmon and Vegetable Kabobs–
–Grilled Chicken Skewers–
–Eggplant Lasagna with Ground Turkey–
–Salmon and Zucchini Noodle with Pesto–
–Stir-fry Turkey and Vegetables with
Cauliflower Rice–
–Grilled Shrimp with Avocado Salad–
–Cauliflower Fried Rice with Shrimp–

✓ Dessert!

–Berry and Coconut Yogurt Bowl–
–Almond and Berries Smoothie–
–Coconut-Almond Dough Bites–
–Baked Cinnamon Apples–

✓ Onwards to Good Health!

What Are You Looking Forward To?

Hey there! Let me share a story with you, an anecdote of change that began in a small town. In this town lived a woman, Alice. She stood at the was in a dilemma of choosing between health and taste, facing the common fight of finding meals that were not only healthy but also seriously delicious.

Fortunately, Alice's adventures took a well deserved turn when she stumbled upon my recipes for lectin-free cooking. And boy, it changed her life! Alice's health story became a live proof of how careful eating can truly make a difference. Frustrated with ongoing health problems, she found herself in a kitchen filled with lectin-free meals that promised not just good health but also amazing taste.

Now, why am I sharing Alice's story with you? Because it's your story too. This guide isn't just about meals; let it be your partner on a trip to better health. It's about enjoying every meal while feeling the positive vibes of a healthy, lectin-free lifestyle.

Imagine starting your day with foods that not only taste amazing but also fill you with energy. Picture lunches that make dull afternoons into delightful experiences, dinners that feel like parties, and treats that fill your sweet needs without compromising on your health goals.

And the best part? It's not just about what you're cooking; it's about knowing the why and how behind lectin-free life. You'll find cooking tips that make your time in the kitchen a joy, nutritional information that strengthens your choices, and flavors that change what it means to eat healthy.

So, here's the go ahead to kick-off on this tasty journey with my recipes as your guide. Your road to healthy living begins right here, in the next pages of the Delectable Lectin-Free Recipes cookbook. It's not just about cooking; it's about recovering your well-being, and I'm here to help you through every step of the way.

Walk with me!

Breakfast!

Welcome to the healthy world of protein-rich, low-carb and letin free meals! Adding these delicious meals to your morning routine can give you a boost of energy and pleasure.

Protein-Packed Scramble

Ingredients:
-3 big eggs.
- Add 1/2 cup chopped spinach and 1/4 cup diced tomatoes.
- 1/4 cup chopped bell peppers.
- Add salt and pepper to taste.
- Use 1 tablespoon of olive oil.

Instructions:
1. In a mixing basin, whisk the eggs until well blended.
2. Warm the olive oil in a pan over medium heat.
3. Sauté tomatoes and bell peppers for 2 minutes.
4. Add the chopped spinach and heat until wilted.
5. Add the whisked eggs and season with salt and pepper.

6. Cook, stirring periodically, until the eggs have set.

Nutritional information (estimate):
- Calorie: 250
Protein: 20g; Fat: 18g.
- Carbohydrate: 5 grams
- Fiber: 2 grams.

Avocado and Smoked Salmon Wraps

Ingredients:
- 1 big collard green leaf (used for wrapping)
- 1/2 avocado, sliced
- 2 ounces smoked salmon
- One tablespoon of lemon juice.
- Add salt and pepper to taste.

Instructions:
1. Lay the collard green leaf flat.
2. Spread sliced avocado over the leaves, then top with smoked salmon.
3. Drizzle with lemon juice, then season with salt and pepper.
4. Roll the collard green leaf into a wrap.

Nutritional information (estimate):

- Calorie: 250
Protein: 15g, fat: 20g.
- carbs: 10g
- Fiber: 7 grams.

Turkey and Vegetable Omelette

Ingredients:
- Two big eggs.
- 1/4 cup chopped turkey breast
- 1/4 cup diced zucchini
- 1/4 cup diced bell peppers.
- Salt and pepper to taste.
- 1 tablespoon of olive oil.

Instructions:
1. In a mixing basin, whisk the eggs until well combined.
2. Warm the olive oil in a pan over medium heat.
3. Add the diced turkey, zucchini, and bell peppers and sauté for 3 minutes.
4. Pour the whisked eggs over the vegetables, seasoning with salt and pepper.
5. Cook until the eggs have been set, then fold the omelet.

Nutritional information (estimate):
- Calories: 280
- Protein: 20 grams.
- Fat: 20g
- Carbohydrate: 5 grams
- Fiber: 2 grams.

Almond Flour Pancake

Ingredients:
- 1 cup almond flour and 2 big eggs.
- Use 1/2 cup unsweetened almond milk and 1 teaspoon baking powder.
- 1/2 teaspoon of vanilla essence.

Instructions:
1. In a bowl, combine almond flour, eggs, almond milk, baking powder, and vanilla essence.
2. To create pancakes, heat a skillet over medium heat and pour the batter in.
3. Cook until bubbles appear on the surface, then turn and cook the other side.

Nutritional information (estimate):
Calories: 120.
- Protein: 5 grams.

- Fat: 10g
- Carbohydrate: 4g
- Fiber: 2 grams.

Spinach and Mushroom Crust

Ingredients:
-4 big eggs.
- 1 cup chopped fresh spinach and 1/2 cup sliced mushrooms.
- 1/4 cup chopped onions.
- Add salt and pepper to taste.
- Use 1 tablespoon of olive oil.

Instructions:
1. In a mixing basin, whisk the eggs until well combined.
2. In an oven-safe skillet, heat the oil over minimal heat.
3. Sauté chopped onions and sliced mushrooms for 3 minutes.
4. Add the chopped spinach and heat until wilted.
5. Pour the whisked eggs over the vegetables, seasoning with salt and pepper.
6. Place the pan in the oven and broil until the frittata is set and brown.

Nutritional information (estimate):
- Calorie: 220
- Protein: 15 grams.
- Fat: 15g
- Carbohydrate: 5 grams
- Fiber: 2 grams.

Coconut Flour and Banana Muffins

Ingredients:
- 1 cup coconut flour
- 4 ripe bananas mashed
- four big eggs.
- Melt 1/2 cup coconut oil.
- Add 1 teaspoon baking powder.
-1/2 teaspoon cinnamon

Instructions:
1. Preheat the oven to 350°F/175°C and line a muffin tray with paper liners.
2. In a bowl, mix the coconut flour, mashed bananas, eggs, melted coconut oil, baking powder, and cinnamon.
3. Mix until well blended.

4. Scoop the batter into muffin cups and bake for 20-25 minutes, or until a toothpick comes out clean.

Nutritional information (estimate):
- Calories: 180
- Protein: 4 grams
- Fat: 12g
- Carbohydrate: 15 grams
- Fiber: 7 grams.

Turmeric and Spinach Wrap

Ingredients:
- 1 big collard green leaf (used for wrapping)
- 2 big eggs
- 1/2 cup fresh spinach.
- One-quarter teaspoon of turmeric powder
- Add salt and pepper to taste.

Instructions:
1. Lay the collard green leaf flat.
2. Scramble the eggs with the chopped spinach, turmeric powder, salt, and pepper.
3. Spoon the scrambled eggs onto a collard green leaf.
4. Roll the collard green leaf into a wrap.

Nutritional data (estimate):
- Calorie: 220
- Protein: 15 grams.
- Fat: 15g
- Carbohydrate: 8g
- Fiber: 5 grams.

Shakshuka and Spinach

Ingredients:
- 2 tablespoons of olive oil
- 1/2 cup chopped onions,
- 1/2 cup diced bell peppers.
- 2 garlic cloves, minced
- 1 tsp cumin and 1 tsp paprika.
- 1/4 teaspoon of cayenne pepper (optional).
- 1 can (14 oz) crushed tomatoes, lectin-free
- 2 cups of fresh spinach and 4 big eggs.
- Salt and pepper to taste.
- Fresh parsley for garnish

Instructions:
1. Warm the olive oil in a pan over minimal heat.
2. Saute the onions and bell peppers until tender.

3. Cook for another minute, then stir in the minced garlic, ground cumin, paprika, and cayenne pepper (if using).
4. Add the smashed tomatoes and bring to a boil.
5. Stir in the fresh spinach and create wells in the tomato mixture for the eggs.
6. Crack the eggs into the wells, cover, and cook until done to your preference.
7. Season with salt and pepper, then garnish with fresh parsley before serving.

Nutritional data (approximate):
- Calories: 280
- Protein: 12 grams.
- Fat: 18g
- Carbohydrate: 20 grams
- Fiber: 6 grams.

Pumpkin and Coconut Flour Pancakes

Ingredients:
- 1 cup coconut flour
- 1/2 cup pumpkin puree
- 4 big eggs.
- One teaspoon of baking powder.

-1/2 teaspoon cinnamon
- 1/4 teaspoon nutmeg.
- 1/4 cup unsweetened almond milk (modify as you like)
- Coconut oil for cooking.

Instructions:

1. In a mixing bowl, combine the coconut flour, pumpkin puree, eggs, baking powder, cinnamon, nutmeg, and almond milk until well blended.
2. Heat the coconut oil in a skillet over medium heat.
3. To prepare pancakes, spoon the batter onto the griddle.
4. Cook until bubbles appear on the surface, then turn and cook the other side.
5. Add your favorite lectin-free toppings.

Nutritional information (estimate):

Calories: 120.
- Protein: 5 grams.
- Fat: 8g
- carbs: 10g
- Fiber: 5 grams.

Of course, you can change these recipes to fit your taste preferences and food needs. As usual, get personalized advice from a healthcare practitioner or qualified dietitian, especially if you have specific health problems or food limits.

Please keep in mind that the nutritional information given is just an estimate and may change based on the exact names or amounts of things used. Adjust amount sizes to match your nutritional needs, and get help from a healthcare expert or chef if you have any special health problems or food limits.

Lunch!

Lunchtime is a chance to refuel your body for the afternoon. These meals can fill you without weighing you down. Here are some ideas for making the most of your lectin-free lunches:

Grilled Chicken Salad

Ingredients:
- 6 oz grilled chicken breast (sliced)
- 2 cups mixed salad greens (spinach, arugula, lettuce)
- 1/2 sliced cucumber.
- 1/2 cup cherry tomatoes (halved)
- 1/4 cup finely sliced red onion.
- 1/4 cup crumbled feta cheese.
- 2 tablespoons olive oil
- 1 tablespoon balsamic vinegar, salt and pepper

Instructions:
1. In a large mixing bowl, add the salad greens, cucumber, cherry tomatoes, and red onion.

2. Sprinkle the salad with sliced grilled chicken and crumbled feta cheese.

3. In a small mixing bowl, combine the olive oil and balsamic vinegar for the dressing.

4. Spread the dressing over the salad, season with salt and pepper, and gently toss to mix.

Nutritional data (estimate):

Calories: 450.

- Protein: 35 grams.
- Fat: 25g
- Carbohydrate: 15 grams
- Fiber: 5 grams.

Salmon Bake

Ingredients:

- 2 salmon fillets (6 ounces each)
- One bunch of trimmed asparagus
- One tablespoon of olive oil.
- Slice one lemon.
- Mince two garlic cloves.
- 1 teaspoon dried dill, salt and pepper

Instructions:

1. Preheat your oven to 400°F (200°C).

2. Arrange the salmon fillets and asparagus on
a baking pan.
3. Drizzle olive oil over the fish and asparagus.
Sprinkle with minced garlic and dry dill.
Season with salt and pepper.
4. Arrange lemon slices on top of the salmon.
5. Bake for 15-20 minutes, or until salmon is
fully cooked and asparagus is tender.

Nutritional data (estimate):
Calories: 450.
- Protein: 40 grams.
- Fat: 25g
- carbs: 10g
- Fiber: 5 grams.

Savory Turkey Skillet

Ingredients:
- 1 pound of turkey,
- 2 spiralized or diced zucchini
- 1 diced bell pepper,
- 1/2 cup chopped tomatoes
- 2 minced garlic cloves.
- one teaspoon dried oregano.
- 1 teaspoon ground cumin

- Salt and pepper to taste.
- Fresh parsley for garnish

Instructions:
1. Cook the ground turkey in a large pan over medium heat.
2. Combine the chopped zucchini, bell pepper, tomatoes, garlic, dry oregano, and ground cumin. Cook veggies until they are soft.
3. Add salt and pepper to taste.
4. Garnish with fresh parsley before serving.

Nutritional data:
- Calories: 380
Protein: 30g, fat: 20g.
- Carbohydrate: 15 grams
- Fiber: 5 grams.

Eggplant and Ground Lamb

Ingredients:
- 4 big bell peppers (halved and seeds removed)
- 1 lb ground lamb
- 1 medium eggplant diced
- One cup of chopped tomatoes
- 1/4 cup chopped fresh mint.

- 2 garlic cloves, minced
- 1 teaspoon cumin
- Season to taste with salt and pepper
- Drizzle with olive oil.

Instructions:
1. Preheat your oven to 375°F (190°C).
2. Cook ground lamb in a skillet over medium heat. Add the cubed eggplant and simmer until mushy.
3. Add chopped tomatoes, minced garlic, fresh mint, ground cumin, salt, and pepper.
4. Spoon the mixture into the halved bell peppers.
5. Drizzle with olive oil and bake for 25-30 minutes, until the peppers are cooked.

Nutritional data (estimate):
- Calories: 400
- Protein: 25 grams.
- Fat: 25g
- Carbohydrate: 20 grams
- Fiber: 7 grams.

Shrimp and Avocado Bowl

Ingredients:

- 8 oz peeled and deveined shrimp
- 2 spiralized zucchini
- 1 sliced avocado, 1 cup split cherry tomatoes,
- 2 tablespoons chopped cilantro
- 1 tablespoon olive oil
- 1 tablespoon of lime juice.
- Salt and pepper to taste.

Instructions:

1. In a pan, saute the shrimp in olive oil until done.
2. Combine spiralized zucchini, cooked shrimp, avocado slices, cherry tomatoes, and chopped cilantro.
3. Drizzle with lime juice, season with salt and pepper, and toss to mix.

Nutritional data (estimate):

- Calories: 380
- Protein: 25 grams.
- Fat: 20g
- Carbohydrate: 20 grams
- Fiber: 8 grams.

Chicken, Broccoli, and Cauliflower bowl

Ingredients:
- 6 oz grilled chicken breast (sliced)
- 2 cups riced cauliflower
- 1 cup broccoli florets.
- 2 garlic cloves, minced
- Two teaspoons of coconut aminos.
- 1 tablespoon sesame oil
- 1 teaspoon grated ginger, and sesame seeds for garnish.

Instructions:
1. In a pan, cook the riced cauliflower, broccoli florets, and minced garlic until soft.
2. Add the sliced grilled chicken to the skillet.
3. In a small bowl, combine the coconut aminos, sesame oil, and shredded ginger. Pour over the chicken and veggies.
4. Stir to mix, simmer for another 2-3 minutes, and serve with sesame seeds.

Nutritional data (estimate):
Calories: 350.
- Protein: 30 grams.
- Fat: 15g
- Carbohydrate: 15 grams

- Fiber: 7 grams.

Cauliflower and Turkey Stuffed Bell Pepper

Ingredients:
- 4 big bell peppers, halved and seeds removed
- 1 pound ground turkey
- 1 cup riced cauliflower
- 1/2 cup diced tomatoes
- 1/4 cup chopped fresh parsley
- 2 cloves minced garlic
- one teaspoon dried oregano.
- Add salt and pepper to taste.

Instructions:
1. Preheat your oven to 375°F (190°C).
2. Cook ground turkey in a skillet over medium heat. Combine the riced cauliflower, diced tomatoes, minced garlic, fresh parsley, dried oregano, salt, and pepper.
3. Spoon the mixture into the halved bell peppers.
4. Drizzle with olive oil and bake for 25-30 minutes, until the peppers are cooked.

Nutritional data (estimate):
- Calories: 380
Protein: 30g, fat: 20g.
- Carbohydrate: 15 grams
- Fiber: 5 grams.

Tofu and Vegetable Stir-Fry

Ingredients:
-14 ounce of firm tofu, diced
- 2 cups broccoli florets
- 1 sliced red bell pepper.
- 1 cup snap peas,
- 2 tablespoons coconut aminos,
- 1 tablespoon sesame oil,
- 1 tablespoon rice vinegar
- 1 teaspoon grated ginger, and
- 2 cloves of chopped garlic.
- Sesame seeds as garnish

Instructions:
1. In a wok or pan, cook the cubed tofu until browned.
2. Place the broccoli, red bell pepper, and snap peas in the pan.

3. In a small bowl, combine the coconut aminos, sesame oil, rice vinegar, grated ginger, and chopped garlic. Pour over the tofu and veggies.

4. Stir-fry the veggies until they are crisp and crunchy.

5. Just before serving, garnish with sesame seeds.

Nutritional data (estimate):
Calories: 350.
- Protein: 25 grams.
- Fat: 18g
- Carbohydrate: 20 grams
- Fiber: 8 grams.

Dinner!

Dinner is the end of your day, and these recipes will provide a satisfying and rewarding experience for a day well spent.

Here are some ideas to improve your lectin-free dinners:

Lemon–Baked Chicken Thighs

Ingredients:
-4 bone-in, skin-on chicken thighs.
- Two teaspoons of olive oil.
- Juice and zest one lemon.
- Mince two cloves of garlic.
- Use 1 teaspoon dried thyme and 1 teaspoon dry rosemary.
- Add salt and pepper to taste.

Instructions:
1. Preheat your oven to 375°F (190°C).
2. In a bowl, combine the olive oil, lemon juice, lemon zest, chopped garlic, dried thyme, dried rosemary, salt, and pepper.

3. Put the chicken thighs in a baking dish and pour the lemon herb mixture over them.
4. Bake for 35-40 minutes, or until the chicken has reached an internal temperature of 165°F (74°C).

Nutritional data (estimate):
- calories: 400
- Protein: 30g,
-fat: 28g.
- Carbohydrate: 2g
- Fiber: 0 grams

Spaghetti Squash Bolognese

Ingredients:
- 1 medium spaghetti squash (halved and seeds removed)
- 1 pound ground beef
- 1 cup chopped tomatoes
- 1/2 cup tomato sauce (lectin free)
- 1/4 cup chopped fresh basil and 2 minced garlic cloves.
- 1 teaspoon dried oregano.
- Salt and pepper to taste.

Instructions:
1. Preheat your oven to 375°F (190°C).

2. Put the spaghetti squash halves on a baking dish, cut side up. Drizzle with olive oil, then season with salt and pepper.
3. Roast the spaghetti squash for 40–45 minutes, or until soft.
4. In a skillet, brown the ground meat. Mix in diced tomatoes, tomato sauce, minced garlic, dry oregano, chopped basil, salt, and pepper.
5. Simmer till heated through.
6. Using a fork, shred the cooked spaghetti squash into "noodles" and serve with Bolognese sauce.

Nutritional data (estimate):
Calories: 450.
Protein: 25g, fat: 30g.
- Carbohydrate: 15 grams
- Fiber: 5 grams.

Grilled salmon and vegetable kabobs

Ingredients:
- Cut 2 salmon fillets (6 oz each) into bits.
- 1 zucchini, cut
- 1 bell pepper, chopped into pieces

- one red onion, sliced into wedges
- Two teaspoons of olive oil.
- One tablespoon of lemon juice.
Ingredients: 1 teaspoon dried dill, salt and pepper to taste.

Instructions:

1. Preheat the grill to medium-high.
2. In a dish, combine the olive oil, lemon juice, dried dill, salt, and pepper.
3. Place salmon pieces, zucchini slices, bell pepper chunks, and red onion wedges on skewers.
4. Brush the skewers with olive oil mixture.
5. Grill for 8-10 minutes, turning regularly, until the salmon is fully cooked and the veggies are browned.

Nutritional data (estimate):

- Calories: 380
Protein: 30g, fat: 25g.
- carbs: 10g
- Fiber: 3 grams.

Grilled Chicken Skewers

Ingredients:
 - 1.5 lbs boneless, skinless chicken breasts (cut into bits).
- Zest and juice from 1 lemon
Ingredients: 2 tablespoons olive oil, 1 teaspoon dried thyme, and 1 teaspoon dried rosemary.
- Season with salt and pepper to taste. - Use cherry tomatoes and bell pepper pieces to skewer.

Instructions:
1. In a bowl, combine the lemon zest, lemon juice, olive oil, dried thyme, dried rosemary, salt, and pepper.
2. Marinate chicken pieces in lemon herb mixture for at least 30 minutes.
3. Place marinated chicken, cherry tomatoes, and bell pepper slices on skewers.
4. Grill for 10-12 minutes, flipping regularly, until the chicken is well cooked.

Nutritional data (estimate):
Calories: 320.
Protein: 35g, fat: 15g.

- Carbohydrate: 5 grams
- Fiber: 2 grams.

Eggplant Lasagna with Ground Turkey

Ingredients: - One big eggplant, thinly cut lengthwise
- 1 lb ground turkey, 1 cup tomato sauce (lectin-free).
- One cup chopped spinach.
- 1 cup almond ricotta cheese (mix almond flour, water, and lemon juice)
- 2 garlic cloves, minced
- One teaspoon of dried basil.
- Add salt and pepper to taste.

Instructions:
1. Preheat your oven to 375°F (190°C).
2. In a skillet, brown the ground turkey. Add the minced garlic, tomato sauce, chopped spinach, dried basil, salt, and pepper. Simmer till heated through.
3. In a baking dish, put the cut eggplant, turkey mixture, and almond ricotta cheese.
4. Repeat the layers and bake for 30–35 minutes, or until the eggplant is soft.

Nutritional data (estimate):
- Calories:420
Protein: 30g; Fat: 25g; Carbohydrates: 20g.
- Fiber: 8 grams.

Salmon and Zucchini Noodle with Pesto

Ingredients:
- 2 salmon filets (6 ounces each)
- Two spiralized zucchinis
- 1/4 cup pine nuts and 1 cup fresh basil leaves.
- 1/2 cup extra virgin olive oil.
- 1/4 cup nutritional yeast.
- 2 garlic cloves, minced
- Add salt and pepper to taste.
- Serve with lemon wedges.

Instructions:
1. In a blender or food processor, mix the pine nuts, basil, olive oil, nutritional yeast, chopped garlic, salt, and pepper. To create pesto, blend until smooth.
2. Season the salmon fillets with salt and pepper. Grill or bake until fully done.

3. Spiralize zucchini into noodles and sauté briefly until soft.

4. Arrange the salmon over a bed of zucchini noodles, sprinkle with pesto, and top with lemon wedges.

Nutritional data (estimate):
Calories: 450.
- Protein: 35 grams.
- Fat: 30g
- carbs: 10g
- Fiber: 3 grams.

Stir-fry Turkey and Vegetables with Cauliflower Rice

Ingredients:
- 1 lb ground turkey
 - 1 grated cauliflower (or processed into rice).
- One cup broccoli florets.
- 1 bell pepper, cut
- 1 cup snap peas and 2 teaspoons coconut aminos.
- 1 tablespoon sesame oil, 1 tablespoon rice vinegar,

- 1 teaspoon grated ginger, and 2 chopped garlic cloves.
- Green onions as garnish.

Instructions:

1. In a pan, brown the ground turkey. Combine broccoli, bell pepper, and snap peas.
2. In a bowl, combine the coconut aminos, sesame oil, rice vinegar, grated ginger, and chopped garlic. Pour over turkey and veggies.
3. Stir-fry the veggies until they are crisp and crunchy.
4. In a separate pan, sauté cauliflower rice until it is rice-like in texture.
5. Toss the turkey and veggies with the cauliflower rice and sprinkle with green onions.

Nutritional data (estimate):

- calories: 400
Protein: 30g, fat: 20g.
- Carbohydrate: 15 grams
- Fiber: 7 grams.

Grilled Shrimp with Avocado Salad

Ingredients:
- 8 oz peeled and deveined shrimp
- 4 cups mixed salad greens (arugula, spinach, lettuce)
- 1 sliced avocado.
- One cup cherry tomatoes, halved
- 1/4 cup sliced red onion,
- 2 tablespoons olive oil,
- 1 tablespoon balsamic vinegar,
- 1 teaspoon Dijon mustard,
- salt and pepper to taste.

Instructions:
1. Grill the shrimp until cooked.
2. In a large bowl, add mixed salad greens, sliced avocado, cherry tomatoes, and sliced red onion.
3. To make the dressing, whisk together olive oil, balsamic vinegar, Dijon mustard, salt, and pepper.
4. Combine the salad and the grilled shrimp, then sprinkle with the mixed sauce.

Nutritional data (estimate):
- Calories: 380
- Protein: 25 grams.
- Fat: 25g
- Carbohydrate: 15 grams
- Fiber: 8 grams.

Cauliflower Fried Rice with Shrimp

Ingredients:
- 1 lb peeled and deveined shrimp
- 1 head of cauliflower shredded or made into rice.
- 1 cup chopped broccoli florets
- 1/2 cup sliced carrots.
- 2 garlic cloves, minced
- Two teaspoons of coconut aminos.
- 1 tablespoon sesame
- 2 sliced green onions.
- Add salt and pepper to taste.

Instructions:
1. In a large skillet, saute the shrimp until done. Remove and put aside.
2. In the same skillet, cook the garlic, broccoli, and carrots until soft.
3. Cook cauliflower rice until it achieves a rice-like consistency.
4. Mix in the cooked shrimp, coconut aminos, sesame oil, green onions, salt, and pepper.

5. Cook for another 2-3 minutes, making sure all of the ingredients are well blended.

Nutritional data (estimate):
Calories: 350.
Protein: 30g, fat: 15g.
- Carbohydrate: 20 grams
- Fiber: 8 grams.

Dessert!

Desserts may be both delicious and lectin-free. These recipes can help you meet your sweet desire without jeopardizing your health goals.

Berry and Coconut Yogurt Bowl

Ingredients:
-1 cup unsweetened coconut yogurt.
- 1/2 cup mixed berries (strawberries, blueberries, raspberries),
- 1 tablespoon almond butter, and
- 1 tablespoon chia seeds.

Instructions:
1. In a dish, combine the coconut yogurt and mixed berries.
2. Drizzle almond butter over the top and sprinkle with chia seeds.

Nutritional information:
- Calories: 300.
Protein: 8g; Fat: 18g.
- Carbohydrate: 30 grams
- Fiber: 12 grams.

Almond and Berries Smoothie

Ingredients:

-1 cup unsweetened almond milk.
- 1/2 cup frozen mixed berries (strawberries, blueberries, and raspberries).
- One-half avocado
- One scoop of protein powder (lectin-free)
- One spoonful of almond butter.

Instructions:

1. Blend almond milk, frozen berries, avocado, and protein powder until smooth.
2. Transfer the smoothie to a bowl.
3. If preferred, add a dollop of almond butter and more berries over top.

Nutritional information:

- Calories: 300.
- Protein: 20 grams.
- Fat: 20g
- Carbohydrate: 15 grams
- Fiber: 8 grams.

Coconut-Almond Dough Bites

Ingredients:
- 1 cup almond flour, 1/2 cup unsweetened shredded coconut, 1/4 cup melted coconut oil,
- 2 tablespoons of almond butter
- 1 teaspoon vanilla essence, and a pinch of salt.
- Extra shredded coconut for rolling (optional).

Instructions:
1. In a dish, mix almond flour, shredded coconut, melted coconut oil, almond butter, vanilla essence, and salt.
2. Mix well until a dough forms.
3. Form the dough into bite-size balls. If desired, roll the balls with more shredded coconut.
4. Refrigerate for at least 30 minutes until firm.
5. Enjoy these energy pieces as a filling, lectin-free dessert.

Nutritional information:
- Calories: 80.
- Protein: 2 grams.
- Fat: 7g
- Carbohydrate: 3 grams
- Fiber: 1g.

Baked Cinnamon Apples

Ingredients:
- 4 medium-sized apples (cored and sliced)
- 2 tablespoons melted coconut oil
- 1 tablespoon ground cinnamon
- One spoonful of coconut sugar (optional)
- Top with chopped nuts (walnuts or almonds)

Instructions:
1. Preheat your oven to 375°F (190°C).
2. In a mixing dish, combine apple slices, melted coconut oil, ground cinnamon, and coconut sugar (if using).
3. Place the apple slices in a baking tray.
4. Bake for 20–25 minutes, or until the apples are soft.
5. Garnish with chopped nuts before serving.

Nutritional information:
Calories: 120.
- Protein: 1g.
- Fat: 7g
- Carbohydrate: 17g
- Fiber: 4 grams.

Conclusion!

Feel free to modify these recipes to meet your own tastes and dietary restrictions. Always get tailored guidance from a healthcare expert or qualified dietitian, particularly if you have certain health issues or dietary limitations.

As we walk this culinary journey together, I want you to be at the receiving end of good health. It's not just about the meals; it's about accepting a lifestyle that benefits your body and soul. Through the streamlined variety of lectin-free treats, we've started on a trip of change, led by the spirit of healthy living.

But our journey doesn't end here; it's merely a starting step to a life filled with energy. Enjoy healthy diets that become a love letter to your body, feeding it with the goodness it deserves. Make every meal a party, a medley of tastes and nutrients that echo with the beat of well-being.

Exercise, oh the art of moving for health! It's not a job; it's a dance with your own power. Engage in activities that you love, be it a quick walk, a dance class, or yoga under the morning sun. Feel the joy in each stretch, the power in every step, and let the energy flow through you.

Remember, it's not about perfection; it's about growth. Celebrate the small wins, relish in the joy of a well-cooked meal, and revel in the strength you gain with every workout. Wellness isn't a goal; it's a lifelong journey, and you're at the center of this amazing adventure.

So, my fellow explorer, take what you've learned from these pages and let it bloom into a lifestyle that oozes health. Your body is a temple, and every choice you make is a brushstroke in the beauty of your health. Here's to a life of balance, a music of well-being where every note sings the song of a better, happier you. Until we meet again on this health path, live, blossom, and taste the flavors of your newfound energy. Cheers to your beautiful health!